Targeting Pain

A Practitioners Guide to Relief

Daniel F. Cleary

Published in the United States by:
Hypnosis for Health Learning Center
And
Clearway Communication
P.O. Box 14784, North Palm Beach, FL 33408
(561) 313-1844   Email: dancleary@juno.com
www.danclearyhypnosis.com

<u>Dedications</u>

To the everyday HEROES; my clients and friends,
living their lives and through example, teaching us all,
a deeper appreciation of life.

To my mother Gert, for her patience and humor.

And to O.H. for her persistence and assistance
in getting this done.

"Do what you can.
With what you have.
Where you are."

T. Roosevelt

INDEX

METHODS

TEMPLATES FOR TRANSFORMATION

AUTHOR'S NOTE

I am a trained hypnotist and a hypnosis instructor; I have no formal medical training. The conclusions expressed in this guide are based upon my personal experience living with severe, chronic pains secondary to a brachial plexus avulsion and the insights gained assisting clients for over twenty years.

For the first five years after my injuries I was unable to sleep in the conventional sense; remaining awake for twenty-four to thirty-six hours before collapsing into fitful sleep of three to four hours at a time, awakening in tears. Then I found hypnosis. Within a week I was sleeping six to eight hours a day, discarded most of the medications that I had been taking and reduced alcohol usage. Hypnosis literally saved my life. Since then I have spent over twenty-five years developing more effective ways to access relief and share what I have learned.

This program doesn't promise single-session, life-long relief and yet I have seen that happen as well. This program is about assisting your client/patient to regain a sense of control in life and develop the skills and abilities to live more fully.

Whatever is happening in the life of an individual, perhaps we can all agree that; *when we feel better, we heal better.* Even in cases where the diagnosis may be considered to be terminal, the simple approaches described here can offer great benefit for the individual.

Whether you are a doctor, nurse, physical therapist, hypnotist or an individual assisting a loved one, this program will make a difference in your life and in the life of those you care for.

In my experience, the question of what hypnosis is or is not is often misunderstood. To me and in the context of this program, what we refer to as hypnosis, whether guided by a hypnotist or self-accessed, is a form of communication.

Life is a series of stories and while there are times when the stories we tell ourselves free us, there are times they limit us as well. This program is about rewriting our stories of life in ways that open greater possibilities and joy in ordinary things, making who we become extraordinary.

There are techniques in conventional hypnosis, NLP, and other approaches and they too are stories in their own rite.

Many of the techniques discussed and embedded in this program are effective most of the time, with most people. However, in this program you will discover that the most important technique is the relationships we develop and the flexibility we maintain when assisting others.

A consideration we can explore is while modern medical and psychological developments are at times seemingly magical, science still cannot identify what the experience of life may be for any individual. There are no set answers, no magic bullets. There is only the individual's experience and how they relate their life to the world around them.

We cannot 'FIX' people; we can assist them to live more abundantly and learn to use innate skills and abilities that we all possess, in ways that enhance the experience of life.

Thank you for your curiosity, caring and sense of adventure as you open this phase of exploration.

Dan Cleary

OPENING THOUGHTS

Addressing pain relief and chronic conditions is a topic that we could discuss for years because by definition, chronic conditions continue for years. The impact in the life of an individual living with chronic conditions is what I refer to as Chronic Identity and is perhaps one of the most misunderstood aspects that we can begin to address as we consider this topic.

I find that many practitioners are often more concerned with their abilities to address chronic conditions than the individuals they assist. Perhaps this may be a result of initial training, the stated severity or duration of the condition, or even the prognosis of the diagnosis.

It is vital when assisting people with chronic, painful conditions that we accept a basic understanding:

'THE PATIENT IS NOT THE DIAGNOSIS!'

We are addressing the *__experience__* of the individual, rather than the diagnosis. Whatever the diagnosis or prognosis may be, this simple understanding moves us from the Pass/Fail situation of fixing something that is broken, to the certainty of success, in that every client has the ability to change their perception. **"When we feel better - We heal better!"** The remarkable effect of this simple credo is that clients often improve beyond expectation or explanation.

In my experience most chronic sufferers come to see hypnotists anywhere from two to six years after the onset of their condition. There are exceptions of course and yet, the medical model usually takes as long as two years to thoroughly explore diagnosis and treatment. By the time most clients have lived with their situation for six or more years, most have given up hope of functional relief.

As more and more medical practitioners are becoming aware of the benefits offered with Mind/Body approaches this is beginning to change. By using the simple approaches in this program the practitioner can often assist the individual to change the way they address the situation and interrupt the patterns before they become chronic.

When individuals live with painful signals it often seems that in the moments before sleep, when all outer distractions begin to fade, the signals are most notable, making the transition from wakefulness to sleep challenging. Through time and experience individuals can develop a habit or expectation that makes these moments a time to avoid or shorten. Pushing oneself until overcome by exhaustion or the use of medications or alcohol are common ways to slip beyond those moments more quickly. Unfortunately these methods can also interfere with the quality of rest and limit the restorative powers of our bodies. Simply telling a person who lives with chronic painful sensations to get more sleep is like asking them not to think about the paisley elephant in the living room.

How do we begin to assist these clients? Imagine how it would be if you were to awaken in the middle of the night to use the bathroom and as you shuffle through the dimly lit rooms, you stub your toe. OUCH! See yourself there, hopping up and down, screaming silently into the night to avoid waking the entire house. OUCHOUCHOUCH!

Now as you imagine that instant, notice the rest of your body and you may recognize that the muscles of your back, shoulders, hips and virtually every muscle of your entire body is tensing, even though the ottoman that attacked you is unlikely to strike again. The only area that is actually sending a signal is your toe and yet your entire body carries the message in reaction to those painful signals. When the source of those signals causes the rest of our body to react in a truly threatening situation we are protected; prepared for fight or flight. When the source of those signals is either sending an incorrect signal or the signal no longer gives useful information and fight or flight are unreasonable options, all those other muscles reacting will eventually begin to break down and develop painful signals of their own. The emotional state of unresolved conflict also begins to deplete our energy reserves and the habitual response of living in fight or flight mode robs us of the ability to rest and digest.

Referred pains can become the opening portal toward relief. Individuals dealing with chronic issues often feel that the painful signals control their life and most have lost track of the difference between the actual signals and the referred physiological and emotional reactions. When we assist our clients to notice the difference between the signals they feel, the way they feel about them, and the referred pains that aren't part of the original situation at all, they may experience the return of a sense of control in life. Discovering that they have the ability to make even small changes can have profound impact in their life immediately.

As it happens, the previous paragraphs contain valuable information and resources beyond those stated overtly. When we recognize that virtually every muscle reacts to signals that seem to announce crisis, we can accept that the body has an incredible communication network already in place and functioning. Suppose that we can use that system to announce comfort, joy or relaxation. The message we send can be modified through intent and practice. Also, I have been referring to 'Pain' as 'painful signals' or simply, 'signals.' The word PAIN always hurts. It is supposed to, the word pain is a descriptive part of our survival system and when everything is at its best, pain is a good thing. When the system no longer delivers valid warnings, it no longer serves us. By referring to the mistaken sensations as signals, we begin to objectify them, separating the individual from the signal.

Simple progressive relaxation can provide relief for those referred pains mentioned earlier and yet, the client has come to address 'THE PAIN' and relaxation may seem to be unapproachable. How do we bypass the immovable wall of pain for a client who knows with certainty that it cannot be assuaged? We put the pain on the agenda for later. It seems simple and yet it usually works well.

When a client comes in and we begin to listen to the story of the experience they know so well, we simply say: 'Okay, we'll get to that in a minute but first, so we can discover the most effective ways to address *that* (here again objectifying the painful signal) I'd like for us to play with your imagination for a few moments.' This tells the client that whatever comes next isn't about 'fixing' their pain, which has been tried by many, for years, ineffectively, or they wouldn't be there. This also removes the challenge of pass/fail and tells them that for the moment we will do something else and by the way, that something may be interesting or playful in itself. I wonder how curious you could be to explore your imagination to discover something interesting. This is just the beginning.

What happens next depends upon the moment and the client. We can ask them about their children or grandchildren or wonder aloud about something funny or dear to them. In doing this we shift the awareness from telling us about the pain in their life, to telling us about their joy. In listening to them and watching their physical expression we can often find ways they already know to feel good. When we see them begin to shift in telling us about the things that are important or dear to them, we can covertly develop anchors or assist them to enhance the sensations they express.

Suppose that they smile when describing a grandchild, we might nod, smile and state enthusiastically that there is nothing like the love of a grandchild. (If appropriate, you may touch them on the shoulder or hand as you say this. It is a physical anchor to go with the anchors of smiling and the enthusiasm.) You may add a statement to the effect that it always feels good to think of the example they mentioned and any time they want to feel good, they know how.

Do they have hobbies or interests that we can use as a resource? Their occupation may offer skills and abilities we can use in designing effective relief strategies they can incorporate easily in their life. Remember that taking what they know how to do and doing it differently is generally easier than teaching them a whole new way of doing something. A musician may be able to 'tune out' discomfort, an accountant may determine that investing more energy in the old reactions simply doesn't add up.

What we are doing is developing resource states to use in other ways later. Suppose that we could be aware of our emotional states, which state would you rather be aware of: joy or pain? Okay, that seems to be a no-brainer.

When we evoke joy or laughter and anchor it, then begin to explore challenges and return to joy or laughter and collapse the anchors, we can literally rearrange the way we think about challenges.

Exploring our client's ability to imagine a Safe Place, a Place of Confidence or Resource, is a more formal method of doing the same thing described above with joy, laughter and grandchildren. These are all ways of engaging the client in using their imagination as a resource and can be used in tandem or individually depending upon the client and the level of rapport that we enjoy.

Ask the client to describe their favorite place in nature or a personal spa where everything they see, hear or feel is there by choice and feels good. I suggest that this is a place of their own, where they can be comfortable by them self.

Is there an area of their body (removed from the area that is uncomfortable) that they can notice and allow to be so filled with comfort that it feels wonderful (remember the communication system and how we imagined that if it can send a message of crisis, it could send comfort? Do it now!) Allow the sensations in that area to begin to fade until they can notice that area as though they were watching someone else's hand or foot. In this way we are dissociating from an area that has little agenda of its own and helping them to experience the Mind-Body connection free from challenge.

AND… 'If I can do it there – I can do it anywhere.'

See Glove of Comfort in Templates section.

CORE CONCEPTS

Before we go further in considering the HOW of assisting clients to enjoy levels of relief, let us first address our role in the process and a perspective which allows a greater potential for success.

In accepting our connection with a client we are accepting/defining our own role in the relationship. There are those who speak of 'Practitioner Centered' and 'Client Centered' approaches and they are... well, they are perspectives that have been considered in addressing clients. I think that what we are actually doing is creating a relationship that includes and goes beyond these concepts.

When we recognize in our clients the courage and strength that they embody and realize the true Hero's Journey that is their life, we are more able to accept them where they are and remain present with them. It is always good to remember that as practitioners, we too are on a Hero's Journey: Our relationship with clients is where our paths converge.

When we experience an event that is so unexpected or traumatic that it interrupts our perspective of the world around us, we can easily lose track of a portion of our identity. The death of a loved one, divorce, or a serious diagnosis can sweep away the foundations of who we think we are: the foundation from which our perspectives are based.

In the context of this program, a life threatening diagnosis or a prognosis of life-long unrelenting pain can be devastating. As practitioners, we may encounter clients who are quite literally, in shock even years beyond the moment when the defining events took place.

Those who have the responsibility of speaking with or delivering the news of these situations are required by informed consent, to tell the individual the potential prognosis, side effects of treatment and more. In the telling we can also listen and remember that:

The patient is not the diagnosis.

Whether a client comes to address chronic conditions, a recently discovered disease process, or the results of a severe trauma, the very fabric of their life is at risk of being torn apart. The impact can be potentially devastating. The chaos in those first moments of their experience, the whether and how of recovery, or the potential of end-of-life situations create incredible and individual impacts in their life. Again, consider the Hero's Journey; treat them with reverence, acceptance and honesty.

YOU ALREADY KNOW TRANCE

Would it surprise you to discover that you are already an accomplished hypnotist? One of the most powerful hypnotic inductions ever practiced anywhere, at least in the western world is; **THE WHITE COAT INDUCTION.**

If you are a medical professional who wears a white lab-coat, or you work in any kind of medical or therapeutic center, your patient enters trance when they enter your office or even before. What you say and how you say it, has power and potential because of who you are: an expert in the field of your specialty. The power of your suggestions may vary according to patient perception of where you swim in the food-chain, but you are already entrancing.

This program is intended to guide you to be more aware of how to use this induction to mutual benefit in your practice.

Patient participation and compliance are probably as effective in outcome as any particular therapy: if they don't follow through, they don't get the benefit of your knowledge and skill. It really is that simple and you already know that as well.

<u>LEMON DROP</u>

If the client has difficulty accepting the physiological link between our thoughts and physical responses you can ask them to imagine a lemon:

…See it there in your mind. Perhaps you can imagine that you are in your kitchen and have a lemon in front of you on a cutting board. Roll the lemon with the palm of your hand to soften it and help to release the juices. Now see yourself picking up a good kitchen knife and as you do, begin to safely slice through the lemon. As the blade pierces the skin of the lemon there is that spray of juices that you can smell as you continue to slice through the lemon and then take one half of it and slice it again. Setting down the knife, you can see some of the juice there on the cutting board and perhaps feel the juice on your fingers as you pick it up. Bring the lemon slice to your nose and smell the aroma for just a moment before touching the slice to the tip of your tongue. The flavor explodes and you can squeeze the slice gently as you taste more of the refreshing juice on your tongue.

When the client salivates while imagining this scene, they have practical proof that they CAN change their physiology with their thoughts!

DOCTOR'S ORDERS

Unless a practitioner has specific medical training, the diagnosis and prognosis as medical issues, are irrelevant. Having said this, it is the effect of these events in the perception of the client that is important. Consider the impact of the diagnosis in the life of the client, whether or not the diagnosis or their perceptions of it are accurate.

By law, doctors are required to tell patients the possible side effects of treatments, which are often rare occurrences and yet can be terrifying. The list of fears and expectations is boundless and we can best assist when we listen to what a client has to say. Keep in mind also what is not said: while they may come to us for relief of physical symptoms, the emotional response to those symptoms is at least as important. The impact of the diagnosis may extend far beyond the medical condition: 'Is this a death sentence?'
"What about my family?" "My finances..." "My profession..." "What's next ...?"

Often when a client comes to a hypnotist, it is because the mainstream medical approaches have been exhausted. Doctors are faced with patients that have reached what is referred to as: 'Maximum Medical Improvement' and still experience pain.

Doctors may have to tell their patient: *"You are going to have to live with it."* This is a life sentence to a prison of pain! Thankfully, as more and more medical practitioners are discovering and implementing the benefits of mind/body approaches in their practices, they are now able to add: *"And I can help you to do that…"* which is a reprieve.

Many people adopt the attitude of 'keeping a stiff upper lip:' Grinding Away at the situation while intentionally ignoring aspects that may interfere with the task at hand. This is a resource state (Just Do It!) that has worked to some degree in the past and we can use the ability behind the state in new ways during our time together. (Notice the kinesthetic language in the above description.)

At the same time, we can allow ourselves to remain nonjudgmental in our observations and assistance: Deciding that the client 'SHOULD' have X, Y, or Z as a reaction to the situation, or as an approach to assuage the symptoms of a particular issue or diagnosis, is just as limiting for us as for them. Again, unless medically trained, we do not diagnose, prescribe or treat our clients.

SKILLS AND ABILITIES

Our clients have within all the skills and abilities they require for success in pain relief. Consider that we are assisting with the *experience* of whatever events they have encountered in their life.

When we focus upon the experience rather than the event, we can also remember that the experience includes all the perceptions, misperceptions and expectations that the individual has used in transforming the event to the experience on a personal level. Any misconceptions, fears, anxiety or expectations of continued or worsening pain demonstrate an active imagination at work. This expression of future possibilities is a resource to us as practitioners. When we recognize the skills utilized to get unwanted outcomes, we can help clarify intent, how the process works and resources that they already use. By celebrating and engaging the clients' existing skills with the confidence that they already know the 'HOW' of the process, relief becomes realistic.

The skills we explore together include past experience, beliefs, filters, resources and many other aspects. There may not be conscious awareness of HOW they are doing the things they do yet they are using perspective and imagination to create their experience. Even if seems difficult to recognize the opportunity that resides in adversity we can help them to access and utilize their skills and abilities.

An example: A woman was seeing me about symptoms of IBS as well as other issues. In our first sessions the symptoms of the IBS had lessened to the degree that for several weeks she no longer used either the prescription or over the counter medications that had been a part of her life for years. Then, at the beginning of one session she told me that she had had a 'terrible weekend:' all of her symptoms had returned and she was miserable. I asked when the symptoms had begun and she told me, 'Friday.' I asked: "What happened Thursday?" and watched the light-bulb go on! It turned out that she had received distressing news: (Legal stuff that had been ongoing and not unexpected, or actually threatening, except in the sense that it was family bickering and as such, disappointing.) I put on my very best, thousand-watt-smile and said: "GREAT!" Well, the look she gave me... "What time Thursday did you get the news and what time Friday did the symptoms reappear?" With her response, we concluded that in about twelve hours, six of which she was sleeping, she was able to recreate all the symptoms that she had been free of for so long. I asked her to describe what exactly, she had felt or done when she received the noxious papers and her eyes changed focus as she recalled the moment. After a slight pause she smiled and said that she was hurt by the family bickering and couldn't speak to anyone about it at the time, so she literally 'swallowed' the emotions related to the issue and went about her day as close to usual as she could. Well, it seems that she didn't digest the emotions she had swallowed and realized HOW she had brought about the return of the symptoms.

The realization that she experienced in this process gave her a greater respect and recognition of her ability to imagine and freed her to use that resource more productively in the future.

*See also: **"The Garden of the Mind"** in the Template section for another example of using existing resources.*

CLIENTS ARE PERFECT

When we consider the abilities of our clients, I wonder how you could imagine for a moment, what it would be like, in your life, when you already are whatever you may think of as perfect. Now, as you allow yourself to consider this perfection, you may already suspect that this is a trick question; and it is.

The events of your life however diverse and varied have led you to this moment, reading this page to expand your ability in assisting your clients and to enhance your own life in many ways. Whatever challenges or difficulties you have experienced, you continue to express your curiosity, determination and willingness to go beyond who you have been. Remember that all of this is true of your client as well.

We all make choices and explore different approaches in becoming who we are. Some choices result in outcomes that seem less than perfect, while others exhilarate and elevate us to amazing appreciation of our potential and joy. Some bring with them satisfaction beyond description... others; not so much.

When we remain aware within, of how even the most difficult and painful of experiences are aspects of the life that brought us here, to this moment, we can truly appreciate our perfection.

As you speak with your client remember that theirs too, has been a Heroes Journey of epic proportion and that they have turned to you as a guide for the next steps in their quest.

<u>BELIEFS</u>

Belief systems are learned behaviors and as such can and do change. When we first consider working with clients and how their beliefs may influence the communication we establish, we include our own beliefs.

When we rely upon our own beliefs as 'True' (which is kind of the point of a belief) let us remember that we too, could be mistaken. In fact, that is the belief that I consider my most valuable asset: ***Whatever I believe - I could be mistaken.*** In the context of this program, if I were to believe that a disease must be cured, then anything short of a cure is failure and that doesn't even open the question of what 'Cure' means. If I believe that my clients have the ability to feel better, I then develop greater flexibility to discover how to assist them in doing so.

Reality is not the event
It is our perception of the event.

(If you have a problem with the statement,
See the paragraph above.)

OUTCOMES

Expected outcomes are integral to allopathic approaches and reasonable in the context of 'treating' a disease or identifiable virus, etc. However, when a client comes to us to address an issue, imagining a specific outcome may create unrealistic expectations and limitations.

If our view of relief were 100% we may be disappointed and consider a 50% improvement as a failure, when it is a HUGE improvement. So let us begin to view outcomes with greater flexibility. *(See 10% Solution – p. 39)*

When creating an image of success or how to make changes in our life, the details are important to clarify the desired goal and recognize the process involved toward fulfillment of the desire. Yet when the outcome (or the path toward the outcome) is too detailed we may not recognize opportunity along the way. It is possible to overlook levels of success entirely when we limit our view of what constitutes that success.

Again: ***When we feel better, we heal better***. Trust that in assisting the client to recognize and access a sense of ease in their life, they are better prepared to deal with whatever else happens.

<u>CONTROL</u>

In many cases, when clients have been given a diagnosis or suffered a trauma it is followed by multiple treatments and testing, hours spent in waiting rooms, countless forms to fill out (all asking for the same information) job loss, sleep loss and the list goes on... The sum total of which is a perceived loss of control: the pain/condition/insurance company controls their life.

Even if life before the onset was tough, most would say, *"I want my life back!"* As we begin to assist these people we can help them to recognize the aspects of their life that they do control. Being able to access a recognizable level of relief, even if on a short-term basis can have an amazing effect in all aspects of life.

A Ten Percent Relief
Can Be a One-Hundred Percent Improvement In Life!

PASS/FAIL - EITHER/OR

A common trap that we can encounter is the pass/fail/either/or situation: It works or it doesn't, there is pain or there isn't and if there is, this doesn't work.

When assisting any client we can be aware of how to open the process by degrees, to include more options. **The Ten Percent Solution** is a prime example of this in action. Often a patient will be prescribed an analgesic or treatment and after using the prescription asked if they are still in pain. When answer is 'YES!' often the implication is that the treatment or medication failed and 'What's Next' is explored. However, there may have been a level of benefit that got lost in the process: with fifty percent relief, the question 'are you still in pain' leads to overlooking benefits they have experienced. This is a simplification of the process and yet offers an insight to the idea. The Ten Percent Solution addresses this in greater depth.

Remember to keep options open and look for the benefits that may be hidden in seeming challenges. Listen to the language of the client for self-imposed limitations. When you notice limitations in the language or expectations of a client, explore options rather than 'correcting' them.

TYPES OF PAIN

Before we can address painful signals it is probably worthwhile to explore the types and nature of pain. For our purpose, there are Psychogenic and Physiological pains. There is also the nature of pain: Acute Pain and Chronic Pain.

PSYCHOGENIC:
While this term is out of favor, this is pain without pathology. Regardless of whether there is an overt, recognizable physiological cause; all pain is real:

If it is PERCEIVED it is REAL!

PHYSIOLOGICAL:
This pain is the result of an identified injury or a disease process. We may effectively reduce the interference of this discomfort in our lives while remaining aware of the message to protect the area of discomfort.

ACUTE PAIN:

This is usually of short duration, often associated with accident or injury. The cause of this pain is usually understandable and reflects normal functioning of the nervous system.

CHRONIC

When pain is ongoing, either as a result of ongoing disease, or due to other factors, it is considered it to be chronic.

RELIEF RESOURCES

RAPPORT

PERSPECTIVE

SENSORY PERCEPTION

PAIN AND SUFFERING

PAIN TIMES THREE

HABIT / EXPECTATION

EMOTIONAL IMPACT

ANGER, FEAR, FRUSTRATION

SECONDARY GAIN

MOTIVATION

CHRONIC IDENTITY

TEN PERCENT SOLUTION

LIMITING LANGUAGE

SELF-TALK

SUGGESTION

SELF-HYPNOSIS

RELAXATION

RAPPORT

Have you ever heard someone state that the intention of a session wasn't achieved because they didn't have rapport? I find this a particularly interesting belief: we cannot, -NOT HAVE- rapport; we can have lousy rapport and yet that IS rapport. Perhaps even more interesting would be the perspective that 'good' rapport is necessary for transformation.

Consider the child or adult who lives in a verbally abusive situation. The statements, 'You'll never be good enough, smart enough, etc.' are put forward in a context that simply gushes with 'poor' rapport and yet can be accepted in the moment and beyond to undermine the individual's self assurance. This is the 'Dark Side' of transformational suggestion in action!

So let us consider rapport in the light of our role as communicators and begin to discover ways in which we can utilize whatever we encounter more effectively. We all like people who agree with us, do we not? In my classes I often ask who the smartest people in the world are. You can imagine the width and variety of answers I hear: it is a trick question; the answer is: whoever agrees with us.

Our beliefs, experience and moods will often determine how we respond in a situation. When we first meet people or clients most of us would like to make a good impression and discover new friends. Some clients are nervous, eager, sad, happy or any combination of these and other emotional states. As professional communicators, it is up to us to remain flexible enough to establish a connection with them that is appropriate to the situation.

Imagine you were standing in a field at the edge of a wooded area and heard a child calling out from inside the tree-line, that they are lost and afraid. You could call back and tell them to follow your voice, keep talking and perhaps the child could find their way. Or perhaps you could go into the woods following their voice, take them by the hand and lead them to the path toward home. Both scenarios can be an effective way for the child to find the path and either may be appropriate in the moment. Yet if it were you in distress, which method would you prefer? This is simply one of my favorite examples of rapport. We are the skilled communicators and by using our abilities we can enter the client's world and assist them to find a path toward success.

We will encounter people who have learned to say 'Yeah But...' to virtually any suggestion they hear. Sometimes simply pointing out what they are doing will help them notice the limitations they are imposing upon themselves and there are times that they will continue to do so from habit. When we press a client to change what seems to have worked in the past, we risk creating resistance that can impede communication and lead to failure. There are also times that by stating suggestions which imply failure, they can; 'Yeah - But' themselves into success. Remain flexible.

A person who has been living with chronic conditions may be somewhat jaded about the possibility of finding relief, simply because of their past experience: they have tried many approaches to reduce their discomfort and they haven't found one that worked. They can be quite literally exhausted with 'one more thing...'

How a client happened to come see us is important. If they are here because:

1) They saw an ad or read a story suggesting hypnosis/mind/body techniques may be effective for their issues.

2) A friend told them that they had heard that hypnosis or mind/body approaches are really effective.

3) A friend or another patient in a waiting room told that they had lived in pain for years and in the first session they found relief.

4) Their doctor suggested they would get quick results that would perhaps surprise them; in fact the doctor often recommends patients to this particular practitioner because they seem to get simply amazing results.

The outcome of our work, especially during the first session, can vary in proportion to the authority of the referral and the beliefs of the individual.

When a client comes to me, I seldom tell them what I think hypnosis is or is not. Rather, I ask them to tell me what they think hypnosis may be, this way I can get an idea of their beliefs and expectations. I also use this opportunity to agree with them, even if their perceptions are mistaken.

Suppose their only experience of hypnosis stems from a stage show at the county fair, where they saw someone bark like a chicken. Well, was that entertaining? Are you here today to learn how to bark like a chicken? And yet, that person on stage was so entranced, they were able to bark like a chicken or sing like Elvis and when the show was over they were smiling. Since most of my clients already know how to bark like Elvis or aren't interested in learning those particular skills, I can then ask them what they would be able to do in their life when they can be so focused and intent.

By exploring together the beliefs and expectations of our client we can begin to develop the possibilities that they can experience. When we phrase our suggestions in the context of 'What if...' we can go beyond the actual experience of the client and open the areas of potential for them to explore. What if... also allows for fantasy solutions as well as 'If I had better skills...'

Imagine whatever you discuss as though it were happening to you. Rather than reading a script, develop your own imagination to describe what you suggest for them. When you are reading a script you cannot watch the client response, in watching the way they respond we can develop the aspects to which they seem to relate most easily. I also find that our clients will respond to pauses by finishing our sentences for us at times.

Everything we speak about is a form of story; capture their attention, involve them in the mystery and trust them to discover the resources that serve them best.

<u>PERCEPTION</u>

Perception is how we experience an event; our point of view. Shifting our perception will offer opportunity to shift the way we respond in any given situation.

Hold your arm out in front of you and while making a gentle fist, point your thumb up toward the ceiling. Breathe deeply and as you exhale begin to focus your attention on the nail of your thumb. Notice your breathing and as you continue to focus your attention on the nail of your thumb, gently close one eye. It doesn't matter which eye you close, just close one eye and continue to focus on the thumbnail.

Now in a moment, as you exhale, close the eye that is open and open the eye that was closed. Now open and close your eyes, back and forth as quickly as you can. As you do this, continue to focus on the thumbnail. Back and forth as quickly as you are able and say aloud what begins to happen.

The thumb seems to move, does it not? Yet you know that the thumb didn't actually move; what changed, quite literally, is your point of view. Your eyes are separated by a distance of about the width of your hand and by looking at the thumbnail from each eye individually the thumb seems to move. When we 'SEE' this, we can begin to understand how our point of view; our perspective, can quite literally move mountains.

SENSORY PERCEPTION

Our senses are the gateways to our perception of the physical universe around us and influence the WAY that we relate to the events of our life.

Most will agree that we have at least five physical senses: Sight, Hearing, Taste, Smell and Touch. Whether what are referred to as Extra Sensory Perceptions are to be included at this level is up to you, the reader. For our purpose we will begin with the big five and let your intuition direct other considerations.

We each have skills and abilities and the senses that we notice as our primary awareness will vary to some degree from person to person. Some people have very acute sight; others may have an affinity for things that they hear, while still others feel their way through life. Naturally there are those that have limited hearing or vision to the point of deafness or blindness. For our purposes, we will consider the following with the presupposition of 'normal' abilities of all five senses and allow that when we encounter exceptions to this, the individual will guide us.

The way that an individual describes the experience of their painful signals will often give us a key to assisting them to shift, reduce or eliminate those signals. One aspect that we will do well to notice is that often a person who is primarily visual in their perceptions may have difficulty in relating to the kinesthetic experience of chronic, painful signals. They may literally not be able to SEE themselves free of physical or even emotional pain.

When we listen to the story or description of the clients' experience they may say that they SEE it as a bright red blob in the middle of their back. Which is a great description as far as it goes. We can ask them if it were a different color would the area FEEL differently. In doing this, we begin to cross their perceptual boundaries. Ask; if it had a shape what would that be? If it had a texture, temperature, size, etc. what would they be and if the aspects were to change what changes would FEEL better as you can SEE them taking place now.

Usually making a large size image of discomfort into something smaller will reduce the level of discomfort. Yet I have had situations when the client said that they couldn't change the size at all. This is a good time to reverse the approach with them. In the majority of the cases where a client said they couldn't make a large painful area or shape, shrink or fade away, the client was so used to having therapies and techniques fail that they were unable to go along with the suggestion. I asked them to make it BIGGER and to make it HURT MORE! EEEK! They can believe that it could hurt more and usually did so almost instantly. Many expressed their disapproval of my suggestion and visibly winced at the increase in their level of discomfort. I replied: "Now we KNOW you CAN change the size and intensity, let's find out how to make it fade." These people were very good at learning to reduce their level of discomfort, once they had proof that they could make changes with the way they perceived the area.

PAIN AND SUFFERRING

PAIN DOES NOT EXIST. Whoops! I suppose that you think you KNOW pain exists because you have experienced it. Right? Okay, what you experienced were the signals sent by your body and interpreted in your awareness.

Most people can easily remember a time when they were involved in a sport or similar situation and at the end of play looked down to discover a bruise or cut that they hadn't been aware of during the activity. Upon seeing it, they begin to feel discomfort from the injury for the first time. The mind/body simply didn't have the time or opportunity to process it when it happened.

How we perceive and process the signals can be influenced by the context of the situation: in true Fight or Flight situations, we need to defend or escape to survive, and the mind/body connection can ignore the signals until the threat is past.

No two people perceive the signals we refer to as pain in the same way. For that matter there are times that any given set of signals will be processed differently by the same individual depending upon the circumstance. The difference between pain and suffering is at least partly a matter of perception, intention and context.

When we have an injury (imagine a broken bone or a cut) there is usually a cycle that is predictable and in that predictability we can find the resources to deal with most situations: a broken bone that has been properly set is placed in a cast and for a few weeks there will be the acute pain signals which respond well to analgesics. Another few weeks and the cast is removed, the bone has healed and the painful signals have diminished greatly, only reminding us when we over do use of the area: still protective of us. Six to ten weeks post injury the pain is gone and life goes on. From the beginning we have been told what to expect and when we take reasonable precautions, we heal well with little suffering: we had a freakin' broken bone of course it hurt, but things will get better. Do we suffer? Perhaps there is a bit and yet… refer to the previous sentence. When the painful signals continue or intensify beyond the expected time, we begin to experience suffering at a new level: the end is no longer in sight and that is scary.

PAIN TIMES THREE

When we recognize an old, familiar signal and then go into panic-alert: "Here it comes, I _know_ what happens next!" We begin to enhance the signal with clarity of memory and exacerbate the physical and emotional aspects through fear/expectation (conscious or un-conscious) and increase the pain while decreasing our ability to effectively release or alter the signal in other ways.

"It feels like a three now, at ten in the morning. Last time that it was a three at ten, it went to a seven by noon and then the afternoon was shot so bad that I was curled up in bed, unable to sleep ..." Anything like that ever happen in your life?

You're in charge of what's next, you steer the bike. Would now be a great time to break that cycle?

HABIT – EXPECTATION

Those living with chronic painful signals develop the habit of living with the situation. This is an aspect of Chronic Identity, which we address in greater depth later in this program. The habit of living with these signals is simply learned behavior and can be limiting or freeing depending upon how we deal with the signals.

Imagine that you were one of the individuals living with a chronic condition. You are planning to go out with friends or family for dinner and in preparing you assess how you feel and project what you will need to do to be able to enjoy your evening. You might pack some extra medication or arrange that you can ride with someone else so that if you decide to self-medicate with alcohol that you won't have the responsibility to drive. Perhaps you need to take along a pillow to sit on or brace behind your back to be able to sit comfortably through the meal.

You know your level of rest and relaxation (or tension and fatigue) and you have learned your endurance pattern from past experience so you accommodate and prepare. This is what anyone preparing for an event of expected duration would do and is a reasonable response. Habit and expectation are not limitations, rather they are simply living. What we want to learn by being aware of the cycle is that while we can have expectations based upon past experience we can avoid locking ourselves into suffering based upon those expectations.

EMOTIONAL IMPACT

The emotional impact upon the individual of living with persistent, chronic pain is impossible to gauge; people respond differently to the situations they experience. As practitioners, presupposing what is the 'Right' amount of impact is a recipe for error.

-All pain is real-
-Even if it is imagined-

This is not to say that the pain is imagined. While medical science can be very good in diagnosing, it is entirely possible for an individual to experience painful signals that have no OVERT causation. Further, the cycle of physiological signals and emotional responses can and often does, exacerbate the experience significantly. Even a low-level pain can interrupt sleep and exhaustion can lower the threshold for tolerance, thus creating a spiral effect that leads toward more and more awareness of discomfort.

There is also the frustration and anger that are so often a part of daily life for an individual living with a chronic condition. Daily chores that seem mundane to others can become intensely frustrating: as an exercise for the practitioner, open a can of soup – with one hand. Wash the dishes, again, one-handed. I won't even suggest that you attempt the daily personal hygiene practices with one hand or even with your non-dominant hand. This frustration burns energy and added to a sleep deprived level of energy can have far reaching effects.

Keep in mind that the emotional impact goes beyond the individual; it has a ripple effect throughout every aspect of their life. The friends, family, workplace and more are affected by the chronic experience of the individual. This program is about communication and you can imagine how challenging communication can be when the individual feels that those around them simply do not understand the challenges they face. Then there is the feeling on the part of the individual that they can't speak about their difficulties because, even to their own ears, it sounds like whining. The fact that the effects of the chronic experience do go to all these areas further intensifies the effect upon the individual as well.

When we feel better, we heal better is an adage that is a guiding principal in the work that I do and you may discover that when we remember this simple concept, that what we do and how we do it begins to change.

ANGER, FEAR, FRUSTRATION

Life was supposed to be fair... wasn't it? Well here you are and perhaps in addition to painful signals, you have developed further physical limitations. Anger is often a part of the experience of living with chronic conditions, at least at first. The fear that pain will intensify, last forever, or will end up killing you is typical, even before considering the idea that you can't do the things you used to enjoy or that people will look at you differently (And wouldn't THAT be frustrating!) Being angry takes a lot of energy and while in the short term anger can be a motivator, the long term result is that maintaining tension eventually destroys or erodes the life we have. When we develop and practice stress reducing techniques we can limit the impact of the habit/expectation reactions in our daily life.

SECONDARY GAIN

Secondary gains are a bad thing, right? Wrong! I tell my clients if they aren't getting secondary gains they are really missing out. I don't know if there are thirdendary gains but get them too! Secondary gains are perhaps very misunderstood and often clients will have been told that they are somehow to blame if they are getting them. To me we should always get secondary gains; we work with clients for a variety of reasons, do we not? I have the great privilege of getting satisfaction in the outcomes of my clients, recognition among my peers as an educator, financial reward and more due to the fact that I have lived with chronic signals for over thirty years. I would never volunteer for it and yet it is secondary gain.

MOTIVATION

Clearly, motivation is an important aspect of any change. When we understand the different types of motivation we can implement them toward success.

AWAY FROM

Our motivation is literally what *GETS US MOVING*. Avoiding discomfort is a powerful motivation, as it is a natural aspect of our *Fight-or-Flight* survival instinct which has proven effective in our evolution.

However, when we move away from things we don't want, we lose motivation because as we begin to succeed our level of discomfort begins to diminish. *Away* lacks a destination; how will you know when you get there?

TOWARD

When we define a goal, we become more motivated toward success as we begin to succeed.

Each step brings us closer to our goal. Realizing the benefits of these steps and recognizing each as a landmark causes them to become more interesting and enticing.

TOGETHER

Our awareness of the power and limitations of motivation allows us to utilize the energy and excitement to fulfill our needs (reducing discomfort.)

CHRONIC IDENTITY

Chronic Identity is really the same as any other experience, in that everything that happens in our life, whether real or imagined, is a part of who we are. When an individual lives with particular challenges they will be influenced by their experience. In the case of chronic, painful conditions, especially those accompanied by physical limitations, the individual will discover and develop their resources while dealing with situations that are often daunting.

Remember that these people are heroes and life is a quest. If you have similar experiences you may find that understanding comes easily. If you have never had to deal with such invasive realities, trust them and honor their courage.

TEN PERCENT SOLUTION

In my experience, people come to a hypnotist for pain management only after several other modalities of treatment seem to have failed. Drug therapy was either ineffective or left the client feeling too drugged to maintain the life they desire. Physical therapy may have been too painful: due to the pain (I have not only heard that one, I have said it!). The client may simply choose not to be dependent on drugs for an indefinite period. They come because of the FAILURE of everything else they have tried.

When I see a client for pain management I discuss the life adjustments that they have made and how they believe their life will change when they learn to eliminate their discomfort. I ask how they would feel about leaving the office totally free of pain. Everyone says how wonderful that would be and I tell them I am sorry, but I can't do that. I explain the difference between pain and discomfort and ask if fifty percent relief would have a positive impact on their life. Yes is the usual answer. Now, the deal: What if you could have twenty-five percent relief, fifteen, etc.?

Help the client understand the improvement they can experience at a level they can undoubtedly achieve. Remember, most of these people have been to the doctors, they have had physical therapy, they probably know more about their condition than the other medical practitioners who FAILED to GIVE them relief.

Many clients have become so entranced by a system treating the diagnosis that they expect any relief to come from the outside. When we involve them and they turn within, they will usually get more than expected.

By stating with certainty that together we can achieve ten to twenty percent improvement today and having them be aware of the immediate positive impact that this will have in their life, we create a win-win situation. When clients can believe in getting recognizable relief, they experience immediate benefit.

Relaxation and visualization will give them at least ten to twenty percent relief, any more than that is a bonus; exceeding expectation rather than failing an expectation of complete relief.

With this success, they can more easily accept what you tell them in the future, you become their hero. By turning that response around, reminding them that they did it for themselves, that they are the hero, you have given them the one thing they need most: a sense of control in their lives.

LIMITING LANGUAGE

The words we use and how we use them are perhaps the easiest aspect of our communication to notice. Many trainers will tell you that there are words that are "NO-NOs" "Bad Words" however; I am not one of those trainers. To me words have power and when we notice the effects of the words we use, we can choose our language to suit the situation and in so doing, improve our communication.

Certainly there are words that have a fairly predictable effect: PAIN, almost always hurts. It is a word used to describe an experience and when we encounter the experience we are generally being made aware of something that needs immediate attention: TAKE YOUR HAND AWAY FROM THE FIRE! While few want to be in pain, most appreciate the warning and as such, pain is a good descriptor of a system that serves and saves us in many ways.

As discussed earlier, when the signals no longer serve us, it may be time to change the words we use to describe them. The word 'BUT' is an amazingly powerful word as well. In my opinion it is misspelled; it should usually be spelled: BUTT, because it turns everything that was said before it to CR*P (another well understood word.) So the words themselves have a certain power, next is the authority using the words and the context of the usage.

When we seek an expert opinion on any subject, we are likely to give a certain power or authority to what we are told by that individual, whether they are the mechanic who repairs our car, the lawyer who represents our interests, or the doctors who we consult to address our physical well-being.

Who is the prime authority on the subject of YOU? Well... you are, of course! So how important is **Self-Talk**? Henry Ford is cited as having said words to the effect of: Whether we think we can or can't, we are right. The words we repeat in our internal dialogue are vital to who we become and reflect who we have been.

When we listen to our clients, we can notice the words they use and begin to assist them toward shifting the language they use which may create limitations in their daily life. This isn't a matter of 'Correcting' them, rather we can help them to be more aware of their language use and what the benefits of that awareness can offer in their life.

There are amazing aspects in our language that we may hear and respond to and yet, perhaps not recognize on a conscious level in our practice or even in our daily life. There are the BIG LIMITERS: EVER, NEVER, and ALWAYS. 'When-EVER it rains, my pain is worse...' Is that true? Every time it rains? Have you EVER been in a movie theater and when you went out you were surprised to find that it had rained and you couldn't tell? Okay, being engrossed in a movie is a kind of trance, so if they say YES, remind them that they already know how to use trance.

TIME

"When the pain is gone, I can get my life back…" The statement is conditional and limits the ability to 'get my life back' until the condition is met. That statement also implies that they have no life when they experience pain. Again, is this a true statement? What would happen when the client is reminded that they do have a life and today, in the office we will explore ways to get back the control that seems to have been lost to the pains, pills, doctors or therapies they have been dealing with?

Time is relative: think about how quickly time seems to pass when you are fully engaged in what you are doing and how time seems to drag on, when you are not. When we state: *"The pains that in the past, interfered in your life, are beginning to change now…"* we create a separation in time. This statement doesn't say that the pains are gone; only that they are beginning to change. The inference is that in the future they may not interfere.

<u>SPACE</u>

"Can you tell me how those signals would seem if we put them over there, on the other side of the room for a few minutes?"

"Where would those sensations be if you were able to have them shift to another dimension?"

Spatial displacement, like time, is relative: engaging the imagination of the client is the key to success. Most people know of what I call "Parental Deafness:" how children can be in the next room playing, running and making noise, while the parent can sit quietly and read or have a conversation. If the tone or some other quality in the child's behavior changes and they need attention, the parent knows and responds.

So how could the client treat those signals as if they were noisy children in the next room? If the signals change from the usual, to a message that needs attention, they can be aware of that. Yet in the meantime, they can place the signal in another room of their awareness and enjoy whatever they are doing.

Clients will often correct you on details and when you agree and use what they suggest as the reason something won't work, it can become the blueprint for how it could.

DOUBLE BINDS

Whether you are already familiar with double binds or are interested in learning more about them, you may wonder how you can use them in your work with your clients.

A double bind seems to offer two ways that a thing can or even must be so and while trying to figure out the options offered, overlook the presupposition that must be accepted to choose option A or B: look t the opening sentence. Are you wondering about HOW to use double binds with your clients? Or are you really interested in learning more about them?

When doing any visualizations or other techniques with a client I like to end whatever we are exploring with:

"As you notice these changes taking place, you may wonder if it is because of the suggestions that I have made for you or just connecting with your own inner abilities. It may be one or the other or even a combination of both. As you wonder about that you may be surprised to notice something that you overlooked in the past and find yourself smiling or curious what else you can feel better about in the days ahead as you use your abilities more and more."

Now this little example uses time (in the days ahead), double binds (options for how it is so), expectation (you may wonder...), and all these distractions that seem to need attention are based upon: *"these changes taking place."*

HIDDEN COMMANDS AND AUTHORITY

"Many of my clients have found great success when they BEGIN TO SEE themselves FEELING BETTER... NOW you may also DISCOVER simple aspects that YOU CAN CONTROL your breathing and FEEL BETTER.. NOW just notice your breathing... etc."

Using the authority of '...many of my clients...' is very permissive in that it doesn't tell them what they will experience and yet it describes a process that they can use. To be successful.

I DON'T KNOW

"I don't know how quickly you will notice the changes taking place. It may be in a moment or an hour, or you may notice improvements building day by day or even more quickly... but you can see for yourself as you begin to access your special place more and more..." In this example there is a double bind in how quickly, and authority by saying I don't know, but you do.

MORE AND MORE

"The more you practice these simple techniques, the more quickly you will discover how quickly you can feel better now and the more easily you can do this whenever you want. Now... breathe in and release..." When we equate the more you do this, the more you get that, then we leave the decision up to them. After all, who likes being told what to do?

There are an infinite number of ways to utilize what is happening at the moment and guide the client to explore options. Keeping things simple isn't always easy and yet when we pay attention to the words we use, the context, inflection and tones that we use, we can discover ways to communicate more effectively and assist our clients to discover greater levels of relief in their daily life.

CHECKING OUT LANGUAGE

One of the challenges of becoming more aware of the words we use can be second-guessing our self to the point of interfering with our communication. As it happens, there is a simple way to PLAY our self past the initial obstacles of awareness and second-guessing. I ask many of my clients to practice on 'others.'

Most of us, in our daily life encounter many people we will either never see again or see only in certain circumstances.

Examples may be; the person standing next to you in line, the checker at the register in the grocery store or the clerk in the post office. (I used to refer to these individuals as 'Throw-Away Friends' and a student suggested that perhaps 'One-Time-Use Friends,' might be more appropriate. There is a lesson in that suggestion: the way we use our language is an ever evolving process, we will all-ways have room for improvement, so go out there and begin to talk funny now!)

I suggest that we engage these people and practice listening to what they say. Think about it, the more people who come through their line, the less they are probably heard, or the more likely they are to be surprised when someone actually pays attention. Engage them, listen to the words they use and respond in ways that leaves them feeling better than before you came along.

These people are trained to say something along the lines of: "Hello; how are you today? Did you find everything you wanted?" What would happen when you reply: "I'm GREAT! How are you?" If they respond as though they are tired, you might ask if they are near the end of their shift and wonder aloud whether there is something special they could do; a special treat for themselves or their spouse on the way home. If they seem fresh and energized you might thank them for being there and making your day just that much better with their smile or their patience with all the people they assist through the day.

The point is to listen to what they say and find a way to tweak it so that they feel recognized and appreciated for being who they are. Now the curious thing about asking your clients to do this, or doing this yourself, is that there are side-effects: by listening OUTSIDE of our self we can begin to re-pattern the language we use within and with less second-guessing. Oh and it feels good.

METHODS

"In measuring a circle,

One begins anywhere."

Charles Fort

A NOTE ON METHODS/TECHNIQUES

Any technique we choose as a method of addressing the issues expressed by a client will work wonderfully some of the time and leave opportunity for vast improvement some of the time. The more complicated the technique, the more complicated the solution. **Keep it simple.**

The relationship we develop with our client is perhaps more important than the particular technique employed. Having said that, our flexibility in the use of the techniques we choose allows us the greatest range of adjustment in response to client acceptance or participation. Techniques are simply stories about accessing success. We live in a world of stories and relate within, as well as with the world around us, through the stories we create and tell ourselves and others.

One very effective method, worthy of consideration is: *Ask the client what THEY believe would work*. If they say that having a 'Magic Pill' or being able to 'Turn off the pain pathways' would work, go with that. Whatever the presenting condition or issue, the client has the key to success within.

I ask clients whether they have any experience with hypnotic/mind/body techniques and if so, how successful they had been with those techniques at the time. If they say, "Yes" and indicate that it was a good experience I ask them to describe in detail the induction process used. Usually a client will close their eyes as they describe the scene: I ask them about the environment, the sound of the hypnotists' voice, etc: their description becomes the induction! If the answer is "No!" I ask them to describe that process and tell them we won't do it that way; *"...But what could have been done differently to make it effective..."* could also become an induction.

We proceed by taking whatever the client brings in and using the skills they possess to develop the most effective approach on an individual basis. When the client begins to describe their experience we can rely upon our knowledge of techniques to recognize the language or imagery that mirrors a technique we know. Then we can simply guide them through that process. When the description of the issue does not mirror a specific technique, it still contains the methods and perspectives that they use. Our job at that point is to recognize and utilize their skills for a better outcome.

The following short description of techniques is not intended to be all-inclusive or to constitute formal hypnosis training. Rather, what follows is a general overview of some basic approaches and terminology.

For the purpose of this program, the term visualization refers to any method of perception: sight, sound, taste, smell, feel, however you understand or perceive, is exactly correct... for you.

DIRECT SUGGESTION

Direct suggestion can be effective in most cases although it addresses the symptom rather than the cause of the discomfort. In cases where the cause is easily recognizable, such as trauma this can be an excellent approach. In cases that the cause is undetermined, we may ask the client for inner guidance as to cause. By addressing cause we may achieve longer-lasting improvement.

As you may infer by the term, direct suggestion is simply stating the outcome or effect desired. Yes, there are some basic guidelines for creating effective direct suggestions that we can learn and practice. Essentially, a direct suggestion is similar to an affirmation. A possible difference between suggestions and affirmations is that affirmations are generally designed for the conscious mind, whereas suggestions are designed for the unconscious aspect of our mind.

In my experience both aspects of awareness share a desire for clarity. It is said that the unconscious mind accepts or rejects suggestions in relation to agreement with existing beliefs, while the conscious mind can use reason to accept, if tentatively, a new idea. In this model, suggestions don't have to be reasonable or even grammatically structured if they are in agreement with existing beliefs.

As a part of the intake I guide clients toward a sense of clarity regarding the desired outcome: they don't want, 'NO PAIN' they generally want a return of comfort. We can't have "NOT." The Ten Percent Solution is an example of how this works so well in practice. In assisting clients, I want to develop affirmations that they can take home and play with and base the suggestions that I use in trance upon what we have discussed together.

With this in mind, let us proceed. Suggestions are often most effective when they follow a simple outline. I remember this as **Four P's and a B.**

Present tense:

"I will" and "I can" are always in the future. "I am already able to relax away some of the tensions and feel better now." is in the present.

Positive:

The subconscious mind ignores negative terms. "Don't think of Pink Elephants." Go ahead and try!

Precise:

Are you willing to practice the techniques we explore four days a week, twice a day or only when you feel that you need them? Which way will be more effective for you?

Provable:

In order to appreciate your success NOW, state your goals in terms that allow the recognition of success from the beginning. "I can access ten percent relief now and with practice, I can get more…"

Believable:

This is important. Do you believe you can reduce or eliminate the experience of pain? Yesssss. Anyone can believe a small step. And anyone can take another and another, fortified and enthused by each small success along the way.

RELAXATION

I mentioned earlier the example of stubbing your toe and how the reaction to that creates tension, preparing us for Fight or Fight response. When an individual lives in the F/F mode, the idea of relaxation is soon forgotten. We know that relaxation lowers blood pressure and allows the entire body to heal more rapidly. Tension cannot exist together with relaxation and the tension expressed in the F/F mode also causes our bodies to manufacture adrenalin and other substances that are great to have when running, but interfere with living. Constant tension also interferes with sleep, digestion and many other aspects of daily life. The cause of most disease includes tension. The response to a diagnosis can cause immense tension... well, you get it..

Relaxation reminds us of the control we have within our bodies. Utilizing our ability to relax builds self-confidence, improves our immune system and energizes our entire being. Here again, when a client regains even the smallest sense of control in life, it can have profound effect in every aspect of their being.

Abdominal breathing oxygenates the blood causing the muscles to relax more easily. By instructing a client to breathe in this fashion, then suggesting that they notice how easily they relax, we utilize physical reaction as a convincer of powerful hypnosis.

Now there is an aspect of relaxation that many overlook: *activity can be relaxing*. I suggest an activity that has no purpose beyond enjoyment. Walking, swimming or gardening might qualify, especially in the beginning. A person living with chronic pain may not be comfortable being quiet at first, so the activity can be a good distraction and the endorphins generated in doing something because it is fun are priceless!

While physical activity may not be an option for some clients, MORE activity than they have been doing usually is. The point that I make here is that whatever they do, they should do it for the enjoyment. Walking, swimming, etc. may have Secondary Gains; however doing them because you enjoy the activity is what is important. Activity for enjoyment relaxes the mind and soon the genuine fatigue will allow the body to remember how to relax as well.

I had a client who had been diagnosed with Fibromyalgia and she told me of the many things that she no longer did because of the pains she experienced. I suggested that she begin walking through her neighborhood at an easy pace. The next time we met she said that she had begun walking and noticed the aches from the activity. I asked her how the aches were different from the sensations associated with the diagnosis and she began to tell me of her experience. As she spoke, she began to smile, telling me about the walk. We came to the conclusion that the aches from increased activity actually felt good: they reminded her throughout the day that she was doing things she enjoyed again and would lessen as her muscle tone improved. Those aches became, for her, a badge of courage. As she continued her increased activity she also noticed that she was sleeping better and the discomfort previously associated with the diagnosis continued to fade.

Relaxation is a necessity in life.

SAFE PLACE

Safe Place is one of the names of an inner resource state of calm and peace. I often refer to this awareness as a **_Place of Resource_** or a **_Special Place_**. The name we use is whatever we agree upon with the client. The use of this approach is simple and can be a powerful resource for the individual. I use some variation of this resource with virtually all clients.

To me, this place resides innately within us all: it is where we go in daydreams, prayer, contemplation or meditation. Like relaxation, Safe Place is a vital resource that is often underrated or misunderstood. I use Safe Place as a home-base from which we can explore other aspects of awareness and to which the client can return at any time.

No 'work' takes place in Safe Place. There are pathways or doors leading off in different directions to address whatever comes up in our sessions. As a part of the self-hypnosis training, which is a core aspect of working with my clients, Safe Place is where they find peace, energy and a sense of calm.

Listen to the client during the pre-talk and ask questions that will assist in creating a wonderful place filled with all the resources the client will ever want or need. Remind them that everything is there by permission and their willing choice.

Many people choose a place in nature, but I have had clients who chose a luxury penthouse with unlimited room-service; the environment is up to the individual. I suggest that it is theirs alone; it is after-all, within them.

By establishing a Safe Place as a point from which to pursue other work, the client always has an option of retreat if for any reason they become uncomfortable during more intense aspects of a session.

Through doorways and paths we can proceed to explore the issues that they choose to address. Some examples in the context of this program of the pathways we can explore might be: meeting an Inner Healing Team, addressing fears related to a diagnosis, a control room from which to turn down the painful signals, etc.

The following excerpts are examples to be considered solely as guides. That these or similar scripts have been so effective, for so many, is the result of listening to the client and together crafting the success.

PROTECTIVE SHIELD

... You may feel this profound relaxation in every muscle, fiber and cell of your body... you may begin to notice a glowing healing sensation... As you begin to experience this sensation you may notice that you feel this sensation in one area more than another... Focus your attention on the area in which you notice this wonderful healing, glowing sensation... It may seem like sunlight, or a radiance within you. As you focus upon it, realize that it spreads to every muscle, fiber, and cell of your body... The more aware you are of the wonderful, glowing, healing radiance within, the more rapidly it begins to flow, easily, naturally, to all the muscles, to every cell and fiber of your being... Now let yourself, allow yourself, to be aware of this glowing, healing energy as it spreads beyond the physical limits of your being and radiates from you, protecting you, and drawing toward you, all the health and joy which is yours and which you so richly deserve...

DISCOMFORT AS AN OBJECT

"... See in your mind or imagine that the discomfort has a size and perhaps a shape. You may see it with a particular color. Perhaps that discomfort has a sound... As you begin to see, hear or imagine the discomfort, allow yourself to begin to change the shape... As you focus upon the shape and size, notice that it begins to shrink... As it shrinks so does the effect that it has had in your life... in the past.

By changing any aspect of the object, the client changes the perception of the discomfort. Utilize as many of the senses as comfortable; perhaps the burning, fiery pain may be cooled by breathing coolness into it.

In the following examples, using a series of controls to gradually effect the change keeps the concept believable. Remind the client to reduce the discomfort until they have improvement, knowing that as they utilize their abilities the improvement increases.

Control Valve

"... See the discomfort as it flows from the (arm, leg, etc.) And imagine it as a fluid, perhaps like water in a hose and as it flows toward your mind where your awareness of it dwells, see a valve, and let yourself, allow yourself, to begin to turn that valve toward the off position. Just as you can reduce the flow or even turn off the hose in the yard, you can reduce the flow or even turn off that discomfort. There... Now. "

Light Switch, Circuit Breakers

"... See in your mind or imagine a switch or a series of switches which control that discomfort and see yourself turning off the switches... As you turn them off, notice how wonderful it feels using your abilities to improve your life, easily and naturally."

A dimmer switch or fan-speed controls are devices which are familiar. Utilizing the familiar allows the conscious mind to accept the suggestion. Consider the occupation, interests or hobbies of the client as a resource for options.

Body as a Robot

"... Your body sends messages to your brain and your brain decides what meaning to assign to those messages. You know how to sit, stand, walk and much more. Your body obeys the commands that you send. Tell your body right now, to stop sending messages which no longer serve you as a warning. The ones you know about and no longer require reminders about to live safely and in health..."

Increase Potential of Medication

"...You can see or feel the medication as it enters your system and goes directly to the area in which it is needed. Instantly having its effect and as you notice this, you may wonder if it because of these suggestions or because of your ability to direct all things in your being... It may be one, or the other, or both... It doesn't matter...* as the medication flows directly to the area which needs it and only to that area... allowing all other areas to function even better now, as your health improves and the medication has it's beneficial effect just exactly as it is supposed to and in exactly the correct manner and location..."

(*The above is a use of a double bind: engaging the mind to decide HOW it is true, rather than whether it is.)

<u>Parts Therapy</u>

A part of you might want to spend the day at the beach and yet the part of you that is interested in learning more about pain relief has you reading this program. Both aspects have merit and yet here you are reading. Was there a conflict that you were able to resolve between the two aspects or parts of you that voiced their preferences? I wonder if you could read the program at the beach.

By "discussing" the inner conflicts and discovering the meaning of the behavior, client may be able to alter the behavior and still get the benefits intended.

If the symptom has been employed as a form of protection, realize that it is no longer needed, or alter the method of protection.

Pain may be a form of self-punishment, a reaction to guilt, or even protection from risk or success.

Pre or Post-Surgical Hypnosis

Implementing direct suggestion, relaxation and visualization techniques may assist the client to reduce fears, remain calm, focused and centered prior to surgical or dental procedures.

Reduction of pre-operative anesthetic required and post-operative analgesics may result from the use of these powerful methods. Post-surgical recovery and healing are certainly enhanced often allowing the individual to resume normal activities more quickly.

When discussing the efficacy of these methods, realize that while certain positive results are reported, the evidence is primarily anecdotal. Science has yet to understand and consistently reproduce the effects of mind-body healing. Perhaps what takes place is activation of the placebo effect and that opens the question of whether the placebo effect is just the body using natural healing powers. The result is usually improved health, perception and awareness. We may be most effective by stating these as unlimited, natural potential.

Anything we agree upon will work.
Listen, Use Imagination, Succeed!

TRANCE INDUCTION

Some hypnotists feel that working with a client requires a formal trance induction. Others recognize that even in waking state we have the opportunity to assist profound change.

Throughout this program many, if not most of the hypnotic approaches we employ, can be experienced while in a waking state of trance. However, a client may also benefit greatly with a more conventional hypnosis experience as well. This is especially effective as they begin learning to develop and use these skills through self-hypnosis in the future.

Keep in mind that up until this point in the experience of the client, most approaches have had limited effect on their level of comfort. Also, we can consider the dramatic effect of formal trance: fulfilling and exceeding expectations can be a form of drama. When a client has 'BIG PROBLEMS' they sometimes feel they need 'BIG SOLUTIONS' to recognize transformation.

When we use a formal approach in the office setting and the client responds well, we can then anchor their response and teach them to access the state or awareness quickly and easily, on their own. The 'AhA!' a client realizes, whether through formal or conversational approaches is what matters most; it is the convincer: the drama.

When assisting a client in my practice, I begin, as most would, by gathering information through the intake discussion. In some cases this discussion becomes the induction process and we work primarily in waking trances. Even in the case where the 'AhA!' comes in waking trance, I also use a more formal trance as a way of teaching them the ritual to access the state of awareness they can recognize as beneficial.

Regardless of your professional title, by reading this material you demonstrate a dedication to learning new perspectives to expand your ability to assist the people who come to you for relief.

If you have already studied hypnotic or mind/body approaches and either know inductions or guided imagery, then you know how to guide someone to use their imagination, and experience an altered state of awareness. Some will call this trance, others will refer to the altered state as meditation, it really doesn't matter what we call what takes place, guiding an individual through the process opens new possibility for them.

If you have no previous experience in leading a client/patient to an altered state, remember the message about the WHITE COAT INDUCTION, relax and as you continue to read, imagine that this is going to be easier than you would have guessed and just might prove to be fun as well! Oh, and I suggest that you begin to practice self-hypnosis on a daily basis to expand your abilities.

3-2-1 INDUCTION

The following induction is easy and quick to use as well as effective. I know I don't have to remind you to read it a few times to yourself and see how easily you can remember the basics, as you speak it in your own words with your client. You already know that. Right?

I will put some commentary in parentheses along the way. I also have put some words in bold type to suggest that you may put slightly more emphasis on them.

Excellent. Can you sit there comfortably and begin to relax now?

(The statement above asks: Can you? rather than a command: Sit there. This also could be taken as a challenge: Can you?)

*As you sit there you may notice when you **focus your attention on your breathing** that it becomes **even easier to allow the relaxation to begin** to spread to every muscle, fiber* *and cell of your body. So just **do that now** as you **listen to the sound of my voice** and begin to breathe easily, effortlessly and let yourself just gently drift in your mind to a very comfortable level of awareness, certain that your subconscious mind will hear and remember all that you need to **feel this wonderful relaxation throughout your comfortable, healthy body.***

*Listening to the sound of my voice and focusing on your breathing always brings **comfort, confidence and relaxation.***

(The next passage links to the last and sets up a cause and effect situation: because you can hear the SOUND of my voice... other things will happen. They hear you say it, so the other things WILL happen. Also it uses sounds that may have been distracting as deepeners.)

*Because you can hear the sound of my voice, you also may hear other sounds: in the room or from outside the room you are relaxing in now. All of these sounds assist and allow you to relax in a way that always brings **comfort, confidence and relaxation**. . . The sounds of traffic, the sounds of people coming and going, doors opening and closing . . . all these sounds and more that you may be aware of . . . sounds that in the past may have distracted you . . . now bring a serenity, a* *comfort and you go even more relaxed, confident in your ability to relax now even more than before.*

(When you speak of breathing, watch the client and time your statement to be what they are naturally doing: when you see them exhale, pause until just before they begin to inhale and say: Breathing in... In this way you are pacing them rather than making them feel they have to adjust to you.)

*   **Breathing in...** brings energy and comfort... **Breathing out** releases any concern or impressions from outside . . . as you drift easily and effortlessly to your own special place . . . your safe place. You know exactly where that is in your own self and go there easily **now...** Breathing deeply and easily, you may find that when you breathe in, **comfortable, confident** and drifting now deeper relaxed than before. setting the pattern... **Now.** Allow your body to feel its best, through drawing in the energy and the **comfort that you so richly deserve** and exhaling any tension or concerns. As you breathe in **experience the comfort** and as you **exhale** notice that you can **breathe that same comfort** down to any muscle, fiber, or cell in your Body, Mind or Spirit.*

*   In a moment I will count; "**Three, Two, One.**"*

When I count: **Three...** *allow the muscles of your eyes and your eyelids particularly, to begin to relax. Those little tiny muscles that control your eyelids... are* **so easy to relax.** *We use them all the time and can easily use them to relax whenever we choose now.*

When I count **Two...** *let that same relaxation begin to spread.... across the bridge of your nose, into the muscles of your cheeks and jaw. You may even* **notice** *that as the muscles of your jaw relax, your teeth separate slightly, as you* **breathe deeply.**

When I count **One...** *allow the muscles of your eyes and eyelids in particular, to become* **so relaxed, so comfortable** *that even if you were to try to open your eyes... you find them* **so comfortable, so relaxed** *that they remain closed. Sealed shut with relaxation. And the* **more you try, the more comfortably sealed they remain.**

Excellent! Very good!

(We all like to be told we are doing well!)

As you **hear the sound of my voice** *guiding you to an even more relaxed and wonderfully comfortable place . . . Listen as I count.*

Three... *Let the muscles of your eyes and eyelids begin to relax.* **It always feels good** *to allow ourselves to begin to relax in this way...* **Always feels good** *to access our abilities as you relax your eyelids and notice the relaxation spreading across the bridge of your nose, up across your forehead and scalp, bringing you* **comfort, confidence and relaxation.**

Two... *allow that relaxation to spread to the muscles of your cheeks and let the muscles of your jaw relax as you* **breathe deeply,** *evenly, and comfortably you may notice that your teeth separate slightly as you* **breathe in the energy and comfort you feel** *flowing throughout your body.*

One... *Allow the muscles of your eyes and eyelids in particular, to remain* **so relaxed and comfortable** *that even if you were to try to open them you find them sealed shut. And when* **you are certain that they are this relaxed,** *you can go ahead and try to open them but find them sealed shut. You can try, but the harder you try, the more certainly sealed they become and as they remain sealed...* **stop trying!**

(If the client opens their eyes, say: "Yes, you are in complete control. Now allow the muscles to relax until they just remain comfortably sealed...")

Let that relaxation spread through the rest of your body: throughout the muscles of your neck, down into your shoulders and arms. Allow the ripples of relaxation to run down your spine, bringing **comfort, confidence and relaxation** *to every muscle, cell and fiber of your Body, Mind, and Spirit.*

At this point you can use a progressive relaxation and/or guide them toward Safe Place.

Templates for Transformation

INTRODUCTION TO SCRIPTS

THE GARDEN OF THE MIND

GLOVE OF COMFORT

FINGER PUMP

DANCE OF THE DOUBLE HELIX

CHANGE SANDWICH

REVERSE SPIN

Introduction to Scripts

When we begin to address the imagery and meanings of transformational language used in working with clients, it is natural to want a proven script: something that works.

To me, when I think of scripts I paraphrase the rabbit in the cereal commercial: *Scripts are for Kids!* I can't help myself!

In fairness, scripts can be very useful to the new practitioner and to the more seasoned professional as well. I read scripts - at home, in my spare time.

A well written script will have language patterns developed through years of experience and insights for addressing the issues of our clients with grace and elegance that are, at times, breath-taking. Conversely, a poorly written script will often make clear the pitfalls of practitioners imposing their beliefs or misconceptions upon the client.

What follows are a few of what I call my templates, and they are merely stories. Read them as if they were something told to you by a friend speaking of an event in their life. Remember the story so that when you see a mutual friend (or perhaps a client) you can tell them all about what happened and perhaps wonder if something like that would help the person you are speaking with to discover something meaningful to them.

I have found that talking about a friend or client's success is a way to introduce a style or approach to a client without getting into 'Let's TRY THIS!' (Try is a contract to exert effort before failure- unless you are modeling clothing.)

When the client responds to the story with agreement, (by nodding or similar signals,) we can proceed. If they shake their head, I can say; "I see you wouldn't follow that..." and tell them about another mythical friend as though that had just been an aside. This gives the opportunity to engage them while in conversational mode when any resistance is minimal.

As to resistance, I believe that the client made the appointment, showed up on time, expressing a conscious willingness to make changes and it is my job to be flexible enough in my approach to bypass any unconscious resistance. To me, unconscious resistance can be a matter of maintaining the status quo, control, or any of many other factors. Yet the client is here, has opened themselves to the possibility of transformation and trusted in me to be skillful enough to assist them to find relief. This is further evidence of their status as Heroes! I am constantly honored.

One of the most amazing aspects about people is the ability to find meaning in seemingly ordinary events or ideas. Here is a fun little thing to experiment with in your life over the next few days: On a small piece of paper; an index card or sticky-note, write one or two sentences about an issue that has been on your mind recently. We all have something that we are working on, keep it simple. Fold the paper and put it in your shirt pocket or even in your bra, if you don't have a pocket. I suggest people keep the paper close to their heart, which is usually where the issue connects in life.

That is it. Just place it there and if you happen to take it out and glance at it from time to time, that is fine, if you only notice it when you change your clothes, that is fine as well. When you get ready for bed, place it under your pillow or on the night stand.

As you go through your day, listen to the stories of the people you encounter and you may be surprised to discover someone telling you the special something that will change the issue you have written and carry in your pocket. When you hear a story, ask yourself: "Is THAT the one?" and if not, just go about whatever you normally do through the day.

I often ask my students to do this and amazing as it may seem, they almost always find the story or perspective that shifts whatever they have written. There have been times that I suggest doing the above and later in class, ask students to share a funny or silly story from their own life and then have another student retell the story. I tell them that this is a great way to learn about scripts. They all do well and then I ask them to open their note and consider how the story they just heard or retold, would change the issue of the message they have in their hands. And Voila'! Transformation takes place!

I can't say HOW this works and yet it does. There is a story of a scientist who studies hypnosis and decides to research a particular technique. He begins by stating:

"It works in practice; let me see if it works in theory."

There are many studies and theories about the human experience: they began before my time and will continue long after I am gone. My observation is that for whatever reasons, we like to explore meaning in the events of our lives. This is both a wonderful way to go beyond our immediate experience and a way to limit ourselves to the known causes and effects of our past experience. What would it be like if we could listen more effectively to our own stories and begin to rewrite the parts that aren't as we choose?

When I first studied hypnosis, one of my teachers told me about the power of metaphors: he said he had a book of "Meaningful Metaphors" which he could reference according to the situation, often before actually meeting his client. Then he went on to the next subject. I was at a loss, I didn't have the book of Meaningful Metaphors and honestly, I was concerned with always having the story at hand that would help my client. Then I discovered that the client carries their personal copy of Meaningful Metaphors, if I was willing to listen.

Our natural search for meaning usually finds it. The meanings we find aren't always accurate and yet, I have had clients who call or come by to see me days, weeks, months, even years after we have worked and tell me about their success. They often tell me that something I said made a difference for them and before I can pat myself on the back for the insightful thing I have said, (in at least as many cases as not ;) they mention something that was said in passing.

This is all about communication. The better we get, the more we have to learn. Go out and make mistakes. If you recognize them, you learn, if you don't, you will eventually.

Daniel F. Cleary

Listen to the client; they have whole worlds of insights to share. The message we think is so important can often be overlooked or mistaken and yet the client will find meaning in things we didn't even know we said.

'The Garden' is great for using unrecognized skills. 'The Dance of the Double Helix' is wonderful to address what a client may believe is an inherited trait. Read the stories, change them, play with them and adapt them for your clients and yourself.

The Garden of The Mind

Years ago, I learned from a client the power of using their own stories to create an outcome that freed them to excel. The client was addressing weight issues and at the second or third session she said: "I can't do this! I have no patience!" During our intake she had stated that she liked gardening, so I spoke with her about my incredible knowledge of the subject. I told her that I do all my gardening at the grocery store. The vegetables are always fresh, the flowers are trimmed and there is no dirt. I told her that I was certain gardening was pretty simple (you don't need a college education to do that!) and suggested that it was probably important to put the seeds in the ground and then cover them and water them. Then I would be able to go back into the house and in the morning, like Jack and the Beanstalk, there would be whatever I had planted and it would be fully grown. Right?

Well, let me tell you; I discovered quite a bit about gardening that day. Apparently there is something to do with loosening the ground all around the plant and fertilizing, pruning, weeding, and MUCH more! There is sunlight and shade, temperature, dampness, more trimming, fertilizing, and it takes weeks, months even years to grow some stuff!

When she was finished (and I can tell you that I was particularly tough to teach that day!) I repeated the highlights as I remembered them and she was kind enough to correct me when I misspoke. I had to admit to her that gardening wasn't as easy as I had previously thought. I even conceded that it must take a lot of care and attention to grow what you wanted to have and get the sizes of healthy plants that would best suit the yard and your desires. In conclusion, I wondered if gardening might require a lot of patience and whether she could ever feel that she knew how to grow her body slim and healthy just as she could take an overgrown garden and get it into shape. Her eyes filled with tears of joy and the session was over.

This is an example of allowing the client to access resources they already possess yet haven't recognized in context and use them toward success. I challenged her belief system and got her to tell me HOW she knew to be successful, drawing the most effective story from her experience, that included all the resources she needed to use in creating what she wanted. By telling me how to garden she became involved, passionate and very clear about all the things that would be required to grow her-self slim. Please notice that the story was hers.

GLOVE OF COMFORT

Most hypnotists receive training in the use of Glove Anesthesia during our certification course. Each instructor will emphasize the points they feel are most important and each student will develop their own sense of confidence in using this and other techniques.

Our clients become aware, on at least an unconscious level, of the conviction we hold in the techniques we employ. When we project the certainty of success in our manner, we establish the powerful working rapport that enables our clients to trust in their own abilities, the techniques we use and the process of change. Glove anesthesia CANNOT work if you don't use it, and will ALWAYS work when you do. What follows is a reference for the concept. Read it and use it until you develop your own approach. Each client is different; speak WITH them and LISTEN.

Formal induction is usually not required when you allow your confidence to shine and perhaps remind the client of the comfortable safety and ease that always awaits them within.

See it in your own mind and tell them the story as a curious and wonderful tale.

The areas in **bold type** or CAPITAL LETTERS are areas to accent or emphasize.

Now. In a moment . . . I'll touch your hand.

When I do, just let your FOCUS ON THE SOUND OF MY VOICE allow that all the beneficial suggestions become a comfortable part of you.

Very good

(Begin light-touch; stroking or tapping on the back of the hand.)

Just notice as I touch your hand that all sensation begins to change...

Many people notice a slight tingling sensation here on the back of your hand... or elsewhere, perhaps on your arm or across your face or forehead.

Others begin to feel a comfortable distance perhaps as though all the things and sensations you are aware of were happening to someone else... like in a movie.

You may realize this in your own way.

However you experience this... All the things I do here simply allow you to be more and more comfortable.

You MAY be aware of my touch...

And all that I do just happens as though you were watching it, aware of it... if at all... from a distance.

(The light-touch and slight tapping is partly to create a physical confusion. Avoid a particular pattern by changing intensity, and pacing their breathing and the sound of your voice.)

Imagine, if you will, that this area... from your wrist all the way to your fingertips is in a comfortable glove.

This glove is perfect for you... custom made - just for you and all the area within begins to feel relaxed and so very comfortable.

You may think of it as a glove of relaxation or... a glove of comfort.

Every part of your hand within this glove . . .

Your wrist, the back of your hand and the palm of your hand, even your comfortable fingers, all the way to your fingertips feel this sensation.

This comfortable tingling . . .

And all that I do causes you to feel better and better...

More and more relaxed.

You MAY be aware of my touch... But all that I do just lets you, allows you, to go further and deeper into this pleasant feeling.

(At this point begin to pinch the hand above and in the area of the web between thumb and forefinger. Begin slowly and increase pressure while watching clients' face. A soothing tone is usually beneficial and a continuous patter distracts.)

More and more comfortable...

You may be aware of my touch while wondering what it is that I'm doing.

Excellent! (It is always nice to hear that you are doing a good job, is it not?)

Or you may just GO DEEPER NOW into this very pleasant state of relaxation.

Noticing the comfortable tingling...

Aware perhaps of my touch . . .

And the wonderful sensations you can notice throughout your entire body.

And especially here within your special glove...

Your glove of relaxation . . . Your glove of comfort...

(You may continue or you may suggest that as they emerge from hypnosis that all sensations begin to return to normal, suggesting that :)

You may bring forth all the wonderful sensations and comfortable impressions into full waking alertness, for as long as you choose to enjoy them. Whenever you are ready... Now.

NOTE: When you pinch, create a mark which will remain visible for a few minutes. When the client emerges from the formal trance attract their attention away from the hand until they mention the pinch. Then ask how hard they think the pinch was. The usual answer is "not very." Agree with them saying, "You're probably right. May I pinch you now that you are fully alert?" Then quickly pinch them hard! When they yelp and pull their hand away, ask them to notice that the spot you just pinched is at most a blush, while the mark from ten minutes ago is clearly more evident. This works.

Notice that I use the terms analgesia and anesthesia interchangeably. By definition, however, these are different conditions. Analgesia allows that the client may be aware of touch or pressure while remaining free of pain. Anesthesia is a condition of being insensible to sensation. The difference may be lost with the client and cause unnecessary confusion. Also note that I avoid the words "numb and paralyzed," as these and similar terms may trigger associations of an unpleasant nature.

Naturally, there are infinite variations. You may ask the client to open their eyes while you are pinching them, to see for themselves how effectively they can change perception. When working with my Hypno-Moms, I will often suggest, after the anesthesia is established, that the glove begins to grow, becoming an EVENING GLOVE OF COMFORT.

Whether you use "The Glove" to establish reduction of painful sensations or as a convincer that the client is in trance, use this at least once TODAY. Then use it more often, certain of your ability and theirs.

ADD IN THE "FINGER PUMP"

Okay, here is an example of flexibility. Instead of doing the pinch in the context of the 'Glove' or perhaps in addition to doing it, you can toss in a simple little piece that will serve the client for as long as they choose.

After you establish the glove, simply add in something like the following. I use 'Magic Serum' in this and have used 'Elixir' and feel certain that you will find and use other terms that work with your clients.

.... Then taking all the relief and condensing it into "a magic serum, of exactly the right potency" and placing it all right there in your little finger. And as you do so, just lift and drop your finger, just like the handle on an old type well water pump. And each time you lift and drop your finger, you pump your own special serum to exactly the correct place to allow that great relief, that sense of comfort, to flow and surround that area there, that in the past, sent the signals that used to cause the discomfort you had then, in the past. As you lift and

drop you allow all the natural and powerful personal prescriptions to flow ...then taking all the relief and condensing it into "a magic serum, of exactly the right potency" and placing it all right there in your little finger. And as you do so, just lift and drop your finger just like the handle on an old type well water pump. And each time you lift and drop your finger you pump your own special serum to the exactly correct place to allow that great relief, that sense of comfort, to flow and surround that area there, that in the past sent the signals that used to cause the discomfort you had then, in the past. As you lift and drop you allow all the natural and powerful personal prescriptions to flow...

THE DANCE OF THE DOUBLE HELIX

Imagine, as you relax more and more deeply, an image or awareness of the spiral, double helix that is called DNA. Most of us have seen pictures and heard descriptions of this elegant, twisting image, holding within itself all of the information of the physical reality and structure of our life.

Now, as this becomes easier and clearer in your mind, notice there are sixty-four gleaming points spread throughout this rotating image. Some of these points radiate in a manner that allows you to know that they are currently active and others simply glow with the potential of activity.

As they rotate there, your intuition... your inner guidance ... lets you know... that a natural aspect of these points is that at different times they switch off and on in various combinations to provide the necessary information to all the cells of your body, most effectively dealing with the constantly changing universe of your experience.

Now, there are times that these different combinations may be activated in ways that are mistaken or in reaction to mistaken understandings and now, you can trust your inner guidance to reset these beautiful, changing, radiating points to the most effective setting; enhancing health, vitality and the graceful, natural balance of life.

Just let yourself, allow yourself, at the count of three, two, one. Breathing in deeply with each number and letting go completely between each count, to see, feel or experience the shifting of these many points until you are at the best setting for the present moment in your life. As you experience this, just let yourself drift, in your awareness and accept the natural state of balance and harmony you so richly deserve.

CHANGE SANDWICH

Discovering Delicious Resources Within

Consider a sandwich. What kind of bread would you like most on your favorite sandwich? You know all the flavors and textures on your special sandwich, consider them now. Many people enjoy lettuce and tomato. Those big, red, earthy, summer tomatoes may be some of my favorites. What do you imagine on your sandwich when you consider all the wonderful ingredients of your "House Special?" Think for a moment of where each ingredient is; in the refrigerator, the breadbox, or in the cabinets. Perhaps you will have to go to the store to obtain the best and freshest ingredients to create this satisfying snack for yourself.

When you have brought together all of the ingredients, perhaps you would enjoy a beverage with this special sandwich. Some people prefer to eat outside on a porch or in the yard while others relax and enjoy listening to excellent music in their favorite room while taking extra time to appreciate their sandwich creation. Whatever is easiest and best for you is the way you can relate well to this now. Makes your mouth water doesn't it? Excellent flavors and textures always begin to satisfy and remind us how good things are in life.

Why am I speaking of sandwiches? Because in that sandwich, we have identified a need or desire in our life: satisfying hunger. We then enrich the image of the desire with specific detail: a sandwich fulfills the desire. At this point we compared our wants with our available resources and began to consider what additional resources we had yet to acquire. Then we took the actions to utilize our resources and produce that delicious sandwich. Whatever our goals or desires, this is the model for effective change.

Perhaps you see now how simply powerful we can all easily be when we are ready to expand our abilities. You may also understand how I feel that the best use of our abilities is to share them. Today may bring an insight, the further expansion of awareness or we may find other benefits as we continue to enjoy using these easy techniques. Because we consciously consider and recognize, as well as utilize, our resources, we begin to receive more of the rewards and joys through consciously creating change.

REVERSE SPIN

By: Melissa Tiers, Contact: http://www.melissatiers.com

This is a nice script that I picked up from an excellent hypnotist and dear friend, Melissa Tiers, who lives and practices in New York. If you ever have the opportunity to attend her programs, grab it! I offer this script with her permission.

Keep in mind that 'Emotion' is literally, Energy-in-MOTION.

Notice the feeling, and which way it is spinning inside of the body. Imagine the spinning feeling now outside of the body. Reverse the spin, and bring it back into your body. Remember a time when you had inappropriate laughter (you know, a time when you laughed big belly laughs when you shouldn't have been) or if you never laugh inappropriately; think of a time when you laughed out loud. Make the scene bigger, brighter, happier and more compelling. Throw the laughter into the spin. Now think of someone you love or have loved unconditionally (it could even be a pet). Really get a sense of that love and those good feelings, make those good feelings bigger, brighter, and more compelling. Throw the love into the spin. Now think of a time when you felt very relaxed and peaceful. Hold your left wrist with your right hand. If you are left-handed, do the opposite. (Do it whichever way you see yourself doing it when you want to feel calm without doing this whole process). While you are feeling those relaxed and calm feelings, make them bigger, brighter, and more compelling. Throw those calm and peaceful feelings into the spin. Take a nice deep breath. Release your hands. Notice what's different.

Thank you for your interest and participation in this program: I am honored.

Your patients are honored as well by your caring and dedication.

If you have any questions about this program or training available, please contact me by phone or Email as listed in the front of this book.

In peace,

Dan Cleary

BIOGRAPHICAL INFORMATION

Daniel F. Cleary is an internationally recognized Hypnosis Instructor, Pain Relief Educator and a Master Practitioner of NeuroLinguistics. Dan teaches throughout the United States and Europe. His specialties include pain relief and personal transformation.

Daniel is a faculty member at many of the national and international hypnosis conferences and has provided specialized training for hypnotists, doctors and therapists since 1996. He has been a course director for Pain Week, an interdisciplinary medical conference since 2007.

Dan came to hypnosis as a sufferer of chronic pain. In 1978 he was partially paralyzed as the result of a motorcycle accident. The major injury sustained is a brachial plexus avulsion, which in his case causes a burning, crushing sensation throughout his arm and hand in addition to paralysis.

For five years after the accident Dan was unable to sleep as we generally understand sleep; he then learned hypnosis and within a week began sleeping more regularly. Since that time he has devoted himself to developing and sharing approaches for the relief of chronic conditions. While the chronic pain signals remain, Dan has learned to shift the discomfort and participate fully in life.

Dan is the author of the successful client guides:

LITTLE BOOK OF CHANGE - *a primer to hypnosis*
CHANGING PAIN - *Relief is realistic*

Daniel F. Cleary, is a Life Member of the International Hypnosis Federation, the American Association of Professional Hypnotherapists, and was awarded a Diplomate in Hypnotherapy with the International Medical and Dental Hypnotherapy Association.

Contact Dan at: www.danclearyhypnosis.com.

14891485R00080

Made in the USA
Lexington, KY
26 April 2012